How To Make Your Own Solid Perfume

By
Gene Ashburner

ISBN-13:978-1503150676
ISBN-10:1503150674

Content

How To Make Your Own Solid Perfume............................7
Ingredients That You Will Require 8
  Beeswax 8
  Carrier Oils 9
  Essential oils and Essential Oil Blends.......................9
Equipment That You Will Require...............................10
  1) A container for the solid perfume (see examples
  below). 10
  2) Double boiler to melt the solid base.....................11
  3) Straw / spoon / spatula to mix the perfume mixture
 12
  4) Glass container to blend the essential oils 12
Carrier Oils 13
  Jojoba Oil 13
  Almond Oil 13
  Grape seed Oil...14
  Olive Oil..15
  Calendula Oil 15
Essential Oils 16
  What is the difference between essential oils and
  fragrance oil? 16
  Essential oils, fragrance oils and extracts that work very
  well in solid perfumes:...17
Essential Oil Combinations That Work Well Together 19
  Recipe 1..19
  Recipe 2..19
  Recipe 3..19
  Recipe 4..19
  Recipe 5..19

Recipe 6...20

Recipe 7...20

Recipe 8...20

Recipe 9...20

Recipe 10..20

Recipe 11..20

Recipe 12..21

Recipe 13..21

Step 1 - Blend Essential Oils 23

Step 2 – Make The Base For The Solid Perfume 25

Step 3 – Add The Essential Oil Blend....................26

Step 4 - Pour The Perfume Into The Container............27

Alternative Perfume Aromas 28

Recipe 1 – Honey Tea Aroma 28

Recipe 2 – Cinnamon Coffee Aroma 28

Recipe 3 – Coffee Aroma 28

Option 1: 28

Option 2: 28

Recipe 4 – Chocolate Orange Aroma 29

Recipe 5 – Chocolate Peppermint Aroma 29

Recipe 6 – Chocolate Rose Aroma 29

Recipe 7 Almond Spice Aroma 29

Recipe 8 – Chocolate Jasmine Aroma 30

Making Solid Perfumes Without Beeswax 31

Another Alternative To Using Beeswax 32

Candelilla Wax 32

Carnauba wax 32

Soy wax 33

Coconut Oil As A Base For Solid Perfume 34

Cocoa Butter As A Base For Solid Perfume 35

Tips For Making Solid Perfume 36

How To Make Your Own Solid Perfume

In this book I will teach you how to make solid perfumes. Instructions and recipes included. Learn about the different essential oil combinations that make great perfumes!!

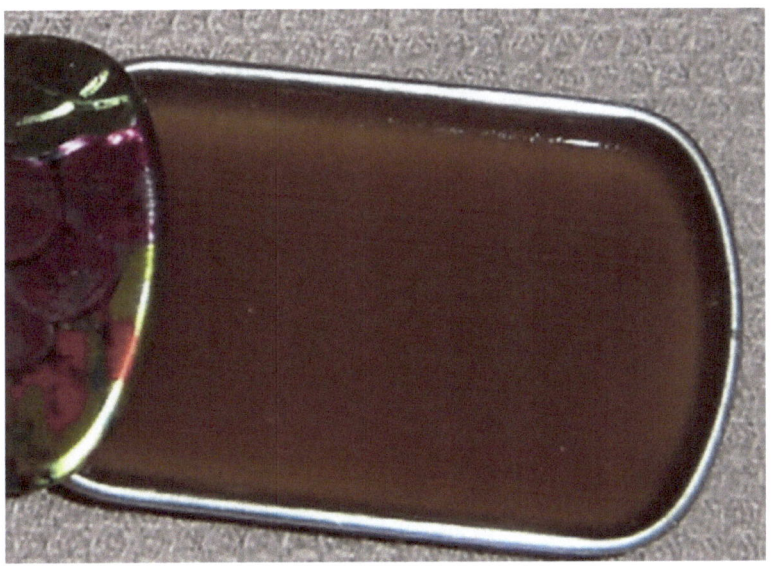

Ingredients That You Will Require

Beeswax

Beeswax (grated or pastilles) OR see the alternatives to using beeswax at the end of this book

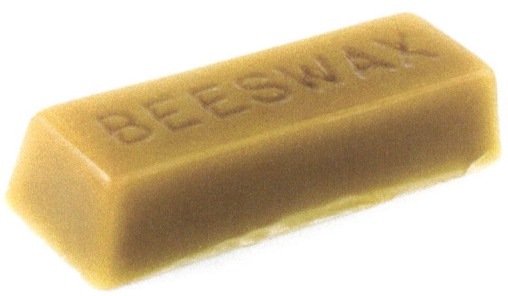

Solid Beeswax

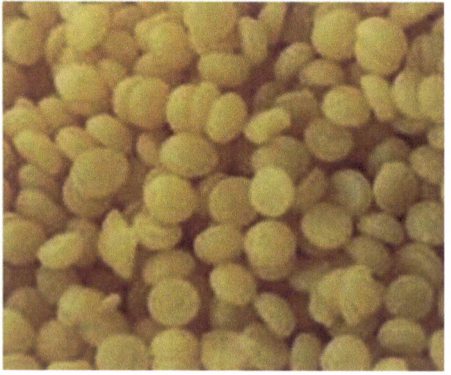

Beeswax Pastilles

Carrier Oils

(see section – Carrier Oils)

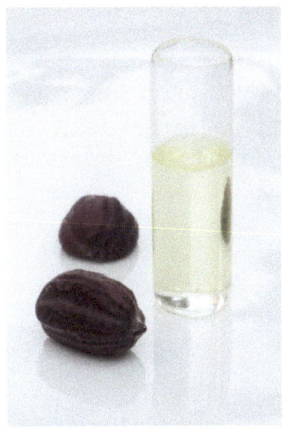

Essential oils and Essential Oil Blends

(see Section Essential Oils)

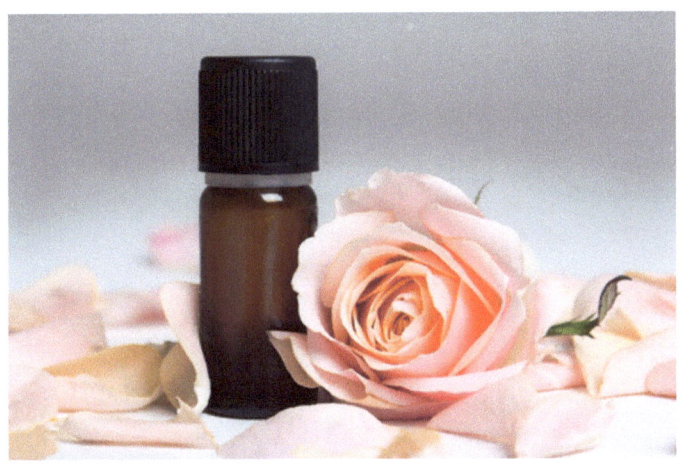

Equipment That You Will Require

1) A container for the solid perfume (see examples below).

You can use containers such as empty chapstick tubes, candy tins, small plastic bottles (with a large opening), trinket boxes and lockets.

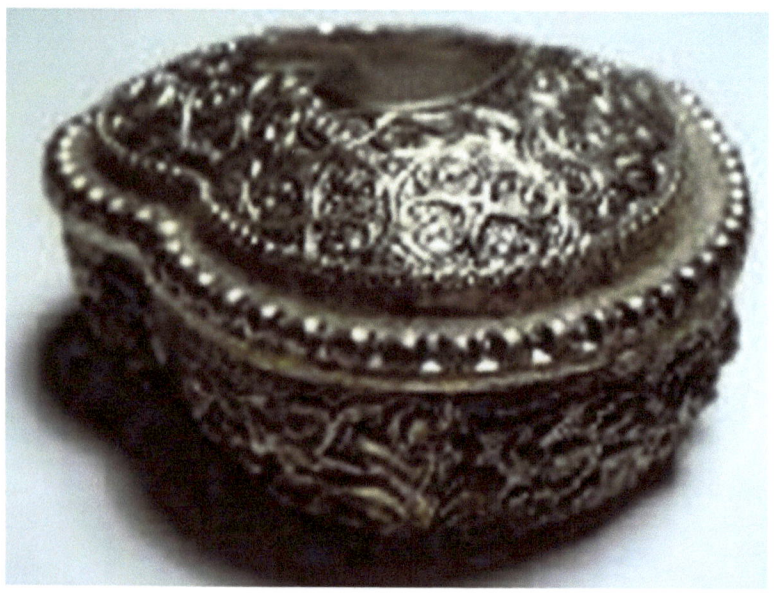

Trinket Box

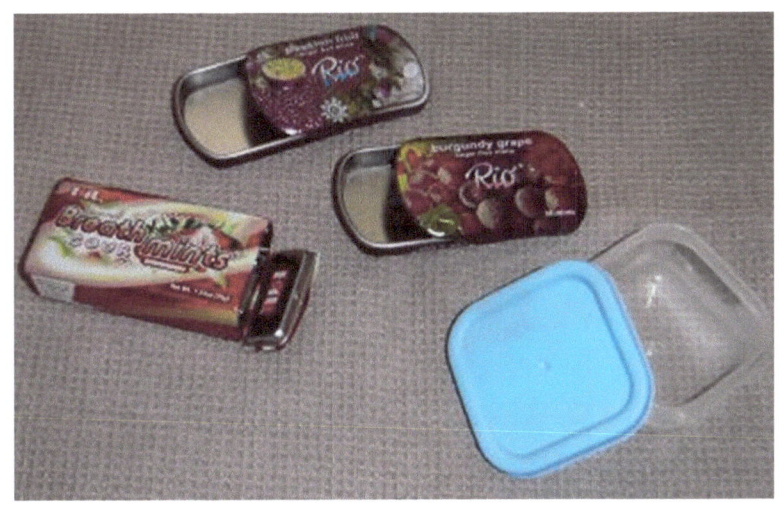

Empty Candy Containers And Small Plastic Containers

2) Double boiler to melt the solid base

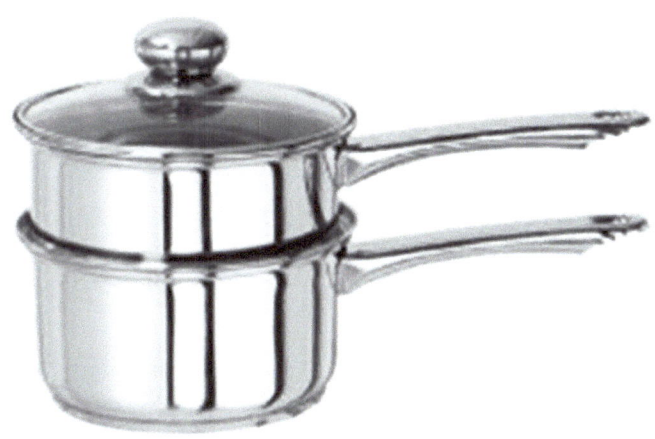

3) Straw / spoon / spatula to mix the perfume mixture

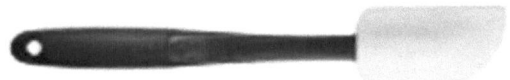

4) Glass container to blend the essential oils

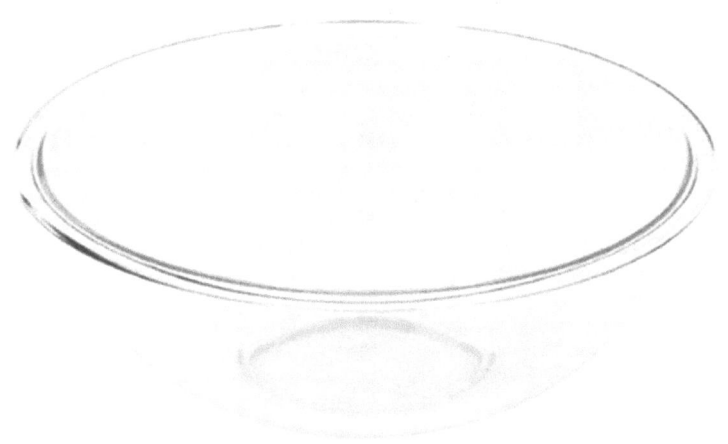

Carrier Oils

Jojoba Oil

Refined jojoba oil is colorless and odorless.

Jojoba oil is safe to use as it can be used on the face, body and hair.

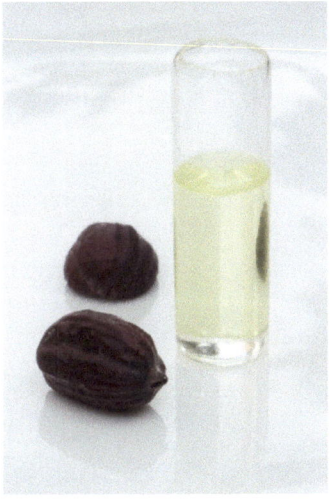

Almond Oil

One gets either sweet or bitter almond oil.

Sweet almond oil has a rich, skin nurturing consistency.

Sweet almond oil provides a very good base for essential oils.

Bitter almond oil is an essential oil and is used for its smell rather than for any other benefits.

Grape seed Oil

Grape seed oil is used in aromatherapy as an all purpose carrier oil.

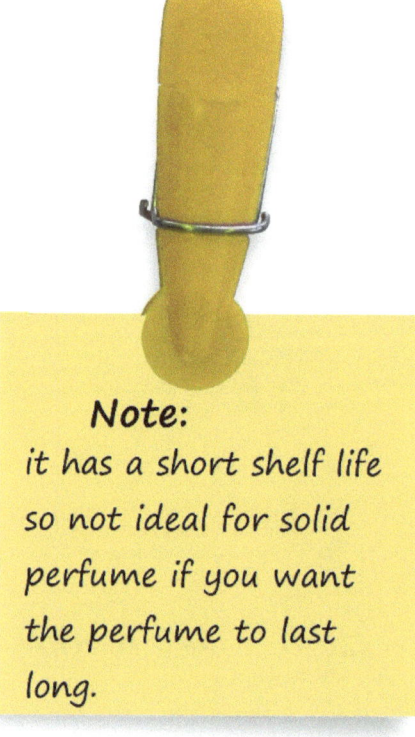

Note:
it has a short shelf life so not ideal for solid perfume if you want the perfume to last long.

Olive Oil

Olive oil is the most universally used carrier oil – it is used both in cosmetics and cooking.

Olive oil has an oily texture and smell and is less preferred than other carrier oils.

Calendula Oil

Calendula oil has great skin benefits and is safe to use in the base of a solid perfume.

Essential Oils

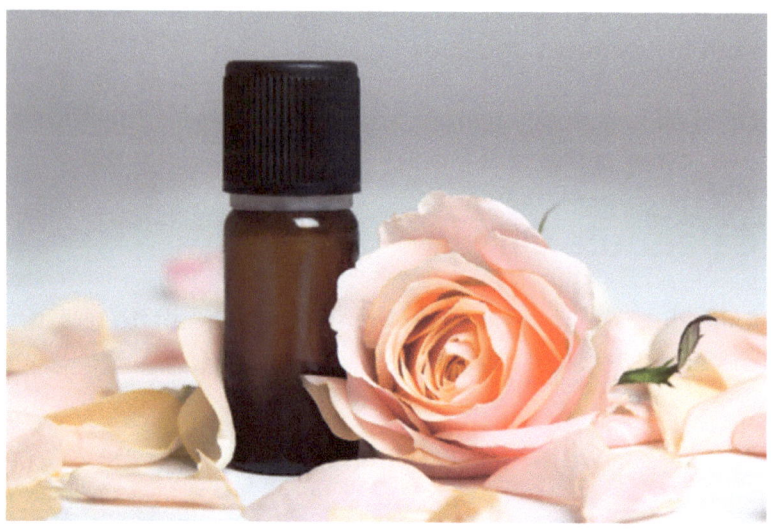

What is the difference between essential oils and fragrance oil?

Essential oils are natural oils.

Fragrance oils could contain synthetics and have already been diluted in carrier oils.

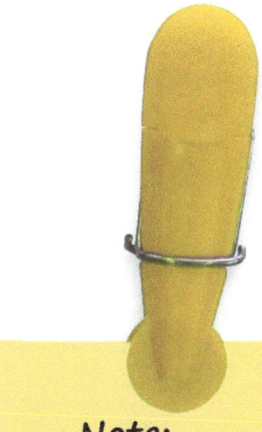

Note:

Not all essential oils are safe for skin use, make sure that you check first before using the essential oil for your solid perfume.

Essential oils, fragrance oils and extracts that work very well in solid perfumes:

- Bergamot essential oil
- Bitter almond essential oil
- Cinnamon essential oil
- Cedarwood essential oil
- Frangipani essential oil
- Frankincense essential oil
- Jasmine essential oil
- Lavender essential oil

- Lime essential oil
- Mandarin essential oil
- Myrrh essential oil
- Nutmeg essential oil
- Palmarosa essential oil
- Patchouli essential oil
- Peppermint essential oil
- Pine essential oil
- Rose essential oil
- Sandalwood essential oil
- Sweet orange essential oil
- Vetiver essential oil
- Violet leaf essential oil
- Ylang Ylang essential oil
- Chocolate fragrance oil
- Coffee Absolute
- Pure vanilla extract

Essential Oil Combinations That Work Well Together

Recipe 1

Sweet orange essential oil
Ylang Ylang essential oil
Sandalwood essential oil

Recipe 2

Bergamot essential oil
Palmarosa essential oil
Pure Vanilla extract

Recipe 3

Patcholi essential oil
Palmarosa essential oil
Pure Vanilla extract

Recipe 4

Bergamot essential oil
Cedarwood essential oil
Ylang Ylang essential oil

Recipe 5

Lime essential oil
Cedarwood essential oil

Recipe 6

Ylang Ylang essential oil
Jasmine essential oil
Sandalwood essential oil

Recipe 7

Frankincense essential oil
Patchouli essential oil

Recipe 8

Rose essential oil
Pure Vanilla extract
Patchouli essential oil

Recipe 9

Jasmine essential oil
Ylang Ylang essential oil
Sandalwood essential oil

Recipe 10

Pure Vanilla extract
Peppermint essential oil

Recipe 11

Sweet Orange essential oil
Bergamot essential oil

Lavender essential oil

Recipe 12

Sandalwood essential oil
Pure Vanilla extract
Myrrh essential oil
Ylang Ylang essential oil
Patchouli essential oil

Recipe 13

Rosemary essential oil
Vetiver essential oil
Pine essential oil
Lavender essential oil
Peppermint essential oil

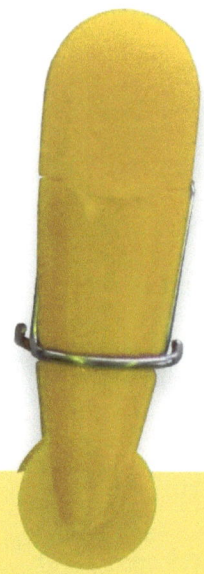

Note:

These recipe ideas are just ideas, you should experiment with different essential oil blends to make up different aromas.

Remember the solid perfumes will smell different on each individual person as the chemical makeup of a person

Step 1 - Blend Essential Oils

Ingredients And Equipment

Approximately 40 to 50 drops of essential oil versus 50 ml of solid base (beeswax and carrier oil mixture)

Glass container

Method

You can either measure out 40 to 50 drops of one essential oil or you can blend different essential oils together in the glass container. See this section for ideas - Essential Oil Combinations That Work Well Together.

Remember to keep in mind that the aroma will mellow once the solid base is added to the essential oil blend.

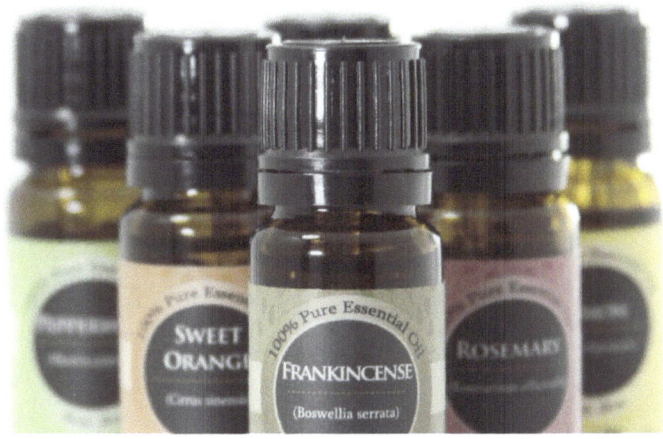

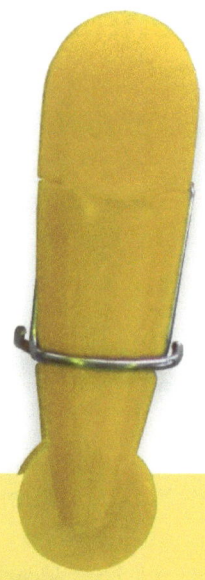

Note:

If the solid perfume is not strong enough once it has been made you can always melt it down again and add additional drops of essential oils. The solid perfume can never be a real disaster!

Step 2 – Make The Base For The Solid Perfume

Ingredients And Equipment

25 ml beeswax (grated or pastilles)

25 ml carrier oil (see section – Carrier Oils)

Double boiler

Water for bottom section of double boiler

Straw / spoon / spatula to mix the melted mixture

Method

Melt the beeswax in the top of a double boiler over boiling water.

Once the beeswax has melted add the carrier oil.

Stir until the mixture is warm and a total liquid.

Step 3 – Add The Essential Oil Blend

Remove the beeswax mixture from the heat.

Add the essential oil blend.

Mix well.

Work quickly so that the mixture does not set before you are done.

Step 4 - Pour The Perfume Into The Container

Pour the liquid perfume mixture into the container that you will be using for the solid perfume.

Leave the perfume to set for about 15 minutes.

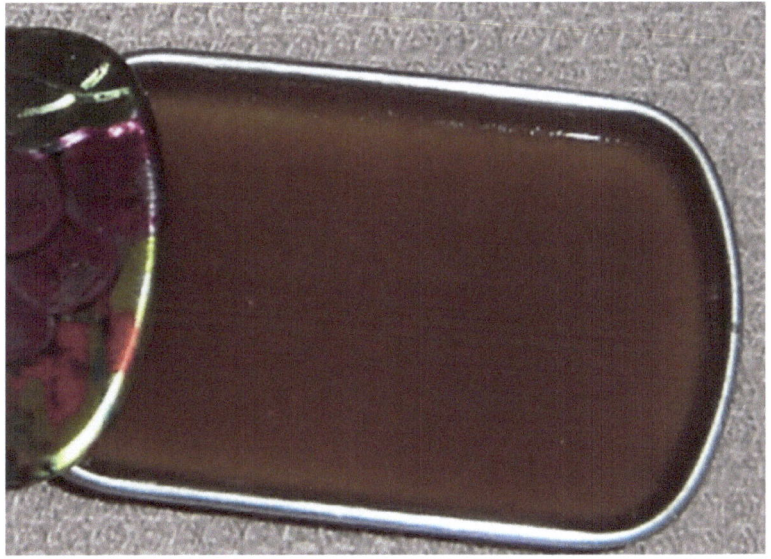

Alternative Perfume Aromas

Instead of using essential oil blends you can make perfumes with the following aromas:

Recipe 1 – Honey Tea Aroma

Pure Honey

Fruit Tea

Recipe 2 – Cinnamon Coffee Aroma

Coffee Absolute (Coffee Absolute is a solvent that is extracted directly from the coffee beans).

Cinnamon essential oil

Recipe 3 – Coffee Aroma

Option 1:

Coffee Absolute (Coffee Absolute is a solvent that is extracted directly from the coffee beans).

Option 2:

Use Coffee CO2 – a fixed oil that has a fatty acid composition and a coffee aroma.

Recipe 4 – Chocolate Orange Aroma

Chocolate fragrance oil

Orange essential oil

Pure vanilla extract

Recipe 5 – Chocolate Peppermint Aroma

Chocolate fragrance oil

Peppermint essential oil

Recipe 6 – Chocolate Rose Aroma

Chocolate fragrance oil

Rose essential oil

Recipe 7 Almond Spice Aroma

Bitter Almond essential oil

Cinnamon essential oil

Nutmeg essential oil

Pure Vanilla extract

Recipe 8 – Chocolate Jasmine Aroma

Jasmine essential oil

Chocolate fragrance oil

Making Solid Perfumes Without Beeswax

Beeswax is not always freely available in some countries and regions, try these options as alternatives to pure beeswax.

Ingredients

25 ml petroleum jelly

25 ml carrier oil such as almond oil

Essential oil blend (your own choice)

Method

The process to make the petroleum jelly solid perfume is exactly the same as the process for making the beeswax version. See steps 1 to 4.

Another Alternative To Using Beeswax

Instead of using beeswax try using Candelilla wax, Carnauba wax or Soy wax. The quantities for the recipe will remain the same as for the beeswax version.

Candelilla Wax

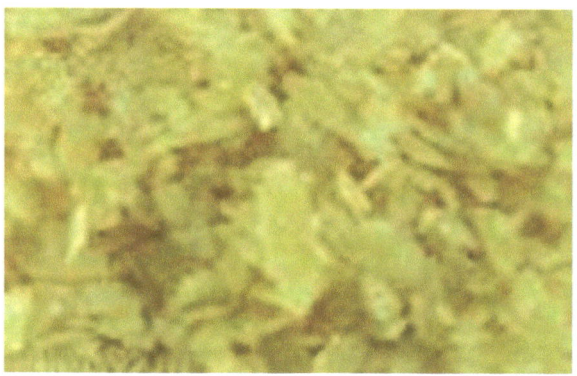

Carnauba wax

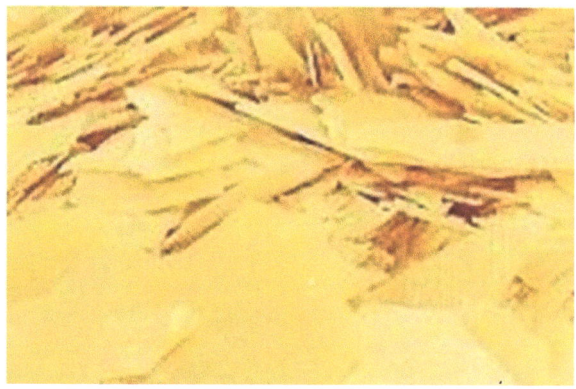

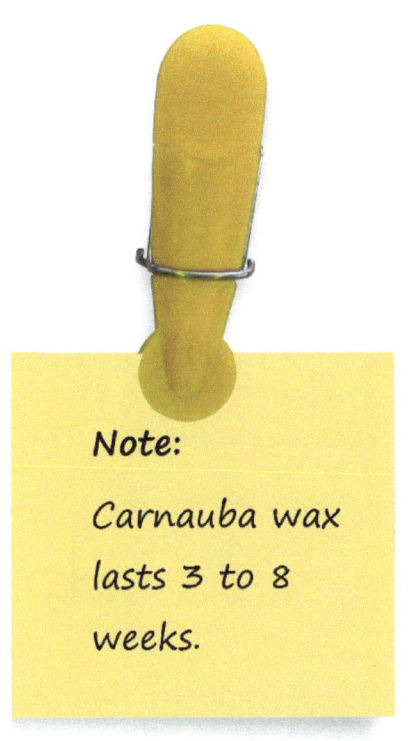

Note:

Carnauba wax lasts 3 to 8 weeks.

Soy wax

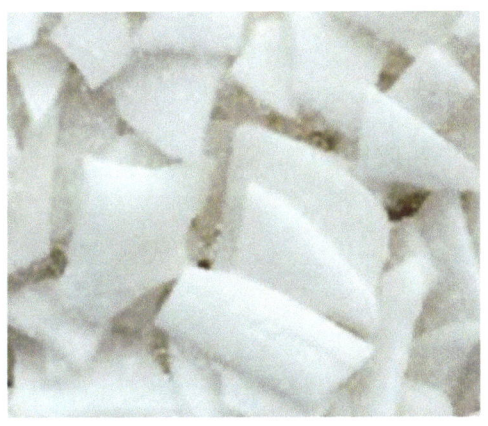

Coconut Oil As A Base For Solid Perfume

Coconut oil stays solid in cool temperatures and melts on contact with skin so it makes a very good base for a solid perfume.

Just be aware that coconut oil melts if it is left in high temperatures. The quantities for the recipe will remain the same as for the beeswax version.

Make sure that you use fractionated pure virgin coconut oil as it has a much longer shelf life.

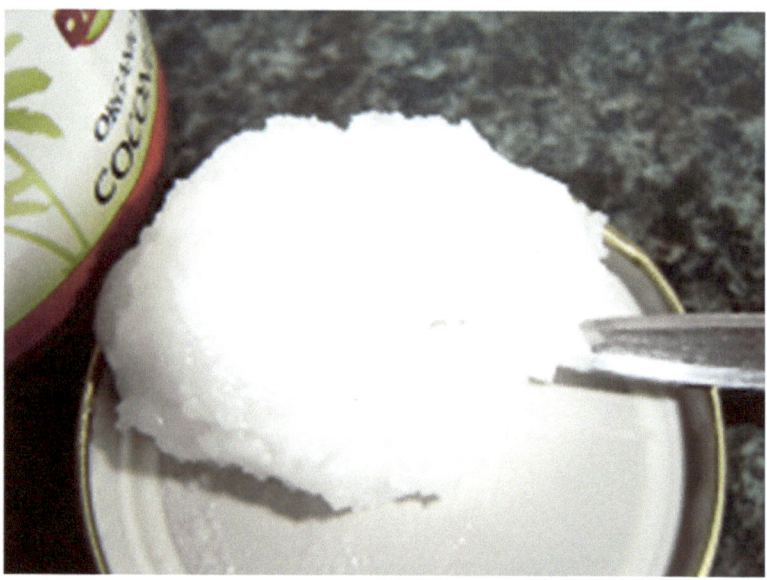

Cocoa Butter As A Base For Solid Perfume

Try using cocoa butter instead of beeswax. The quantities for the recipe will remain the same as for the beeswax version.

Remember that cocoa butter has a strong aroma so take that into account when blending your essential oils, fragrance oils and extracts.

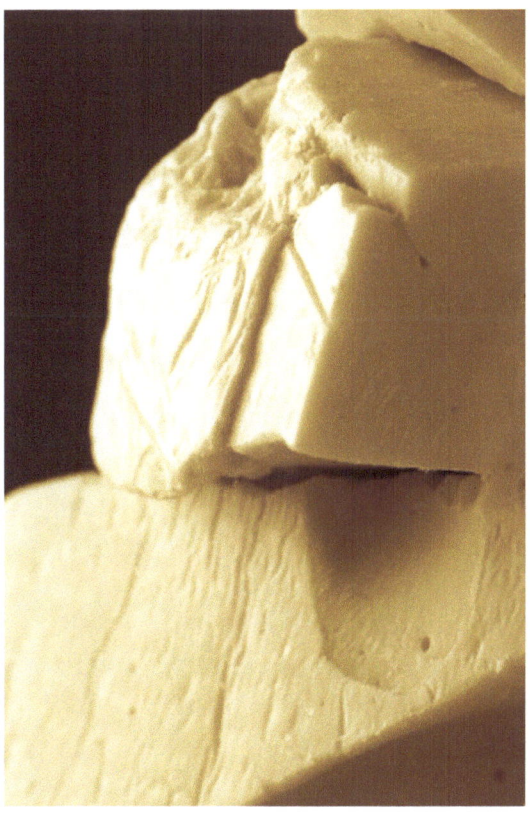

Tips For Making Solid Perfume

If the perfume is too mushy, it means that too little beeswax or beeswax alternative has been used when making the solid perfume. The solution is to melt the solid perfume again and to add more beeswax or beeswax alternative.

If the perfume sets before it has been poured into the container, just reheat the mixture and re-pour the perfume into its container.

Make sure that you add enough essential oil blend as the mixture will tone down the aroma once the solid base has been added, the perfume could end up having too weak an aroma.

Use a bowl that you are not sorry for when you melt the wax, as it is a messy job. Use brown paper to wipe out the excess melted wax and then wash the bowl in the hot water.

Allow the solid perfume to stand for a week or so before using it, the perfume will be much stronger that way.

Use fractionated coconut oil to give the solid perfume a long shelf life.

Remember beeswax has a honey odor and that does not always work well with certain aromas. What are your alternatives if you don't want the honey odor?

See the beeswax alternatives in this book.

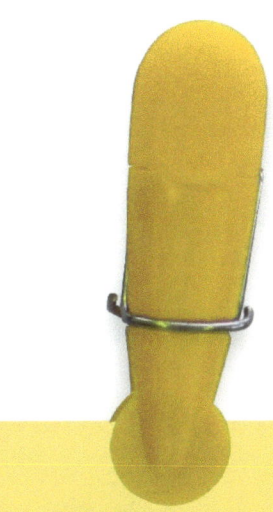

Note:

You can buy filtered, bleached beeswax with no aroma.